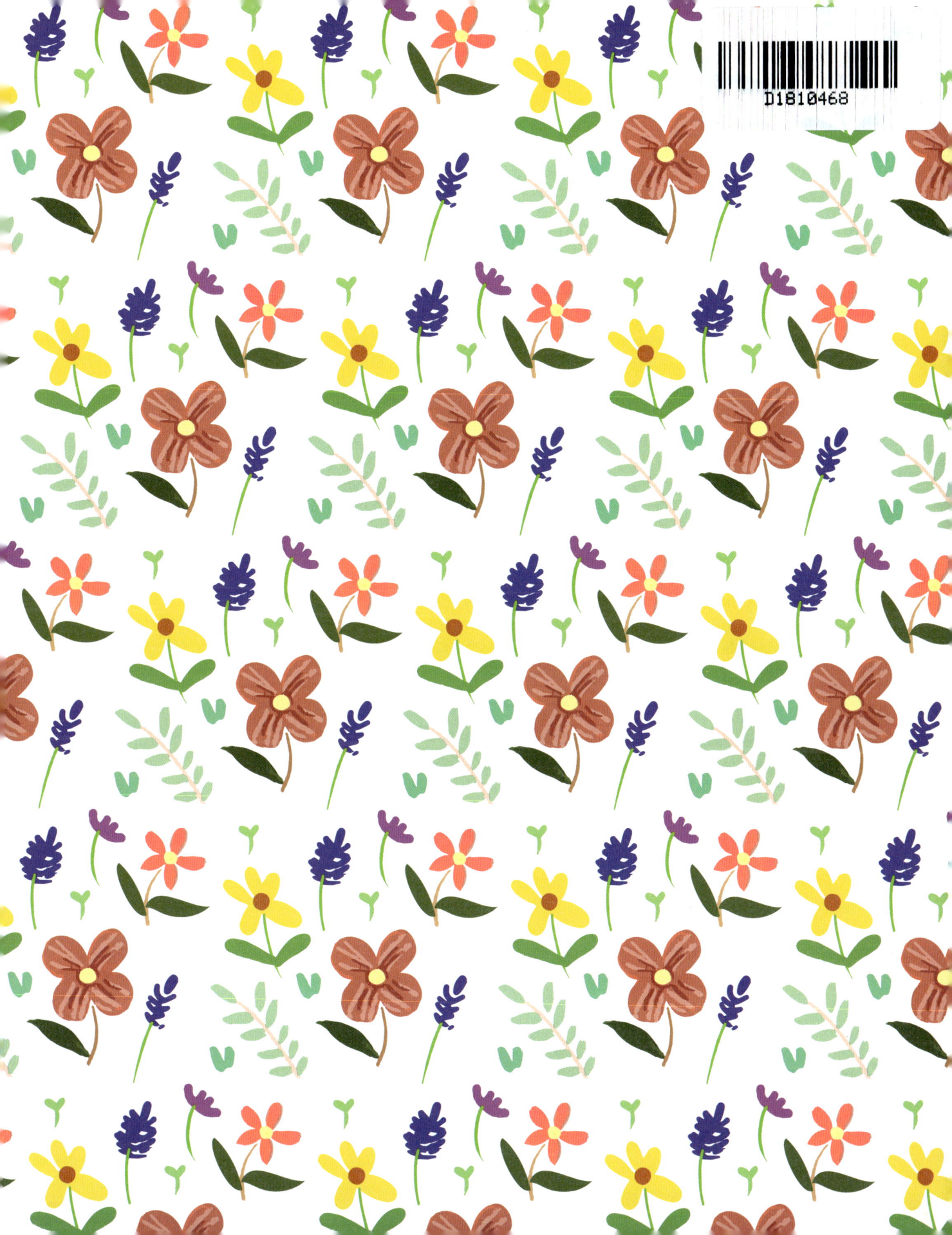

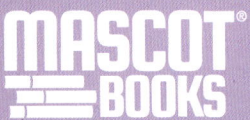

www.mascotbooks.com

You Can Do it, Chickadee

For more information, please contact:
Mascot Books
620 Herndon Parkway, Suite 320
Herndon, VA 20170
info@mascotbooks.com

Library of Congress Control Number: 2020918725

CPSIA Code: PRT1120A
ISBN-13: 978-1-64543-688-1

Printed in the United States

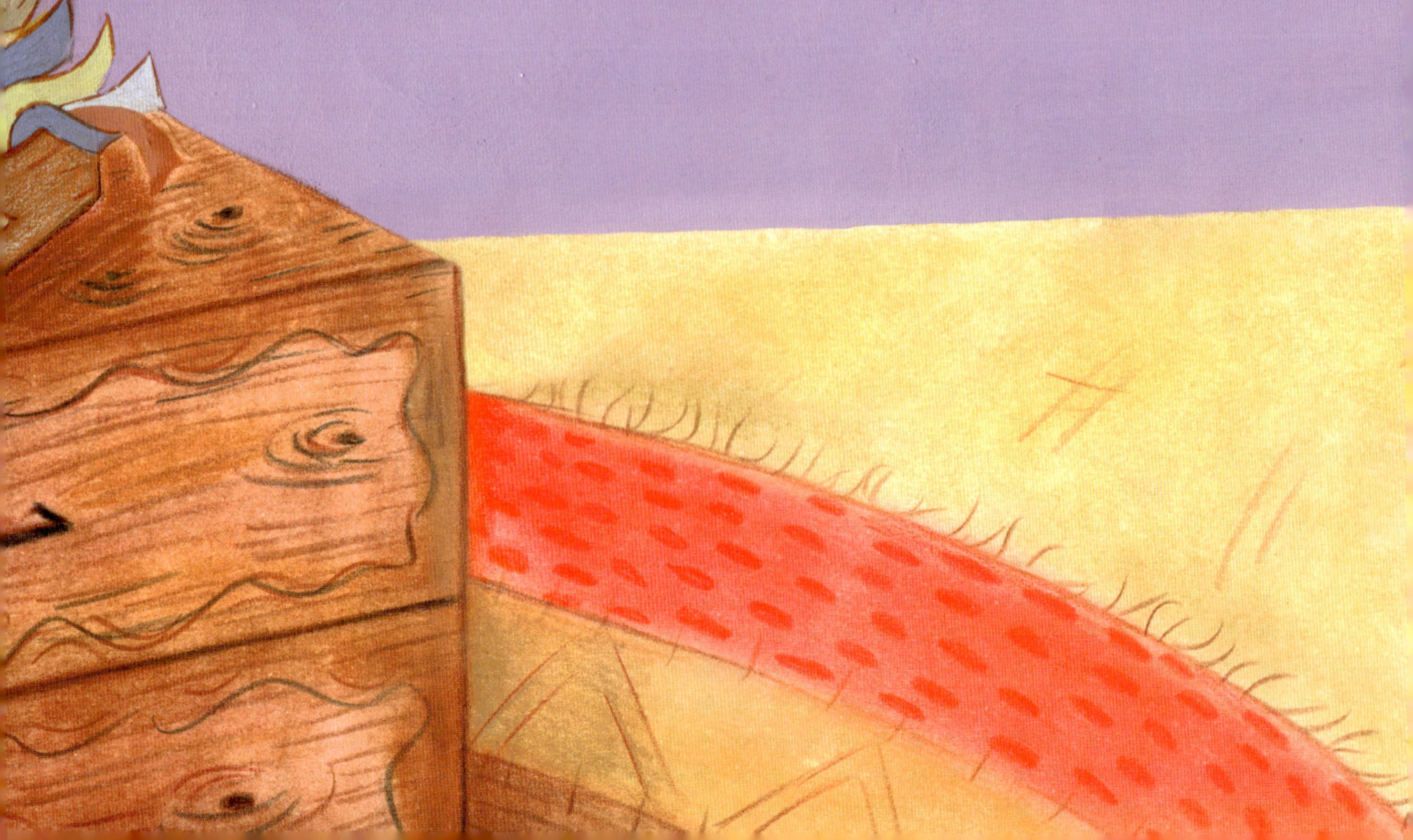

You Can Do it, Chickadee

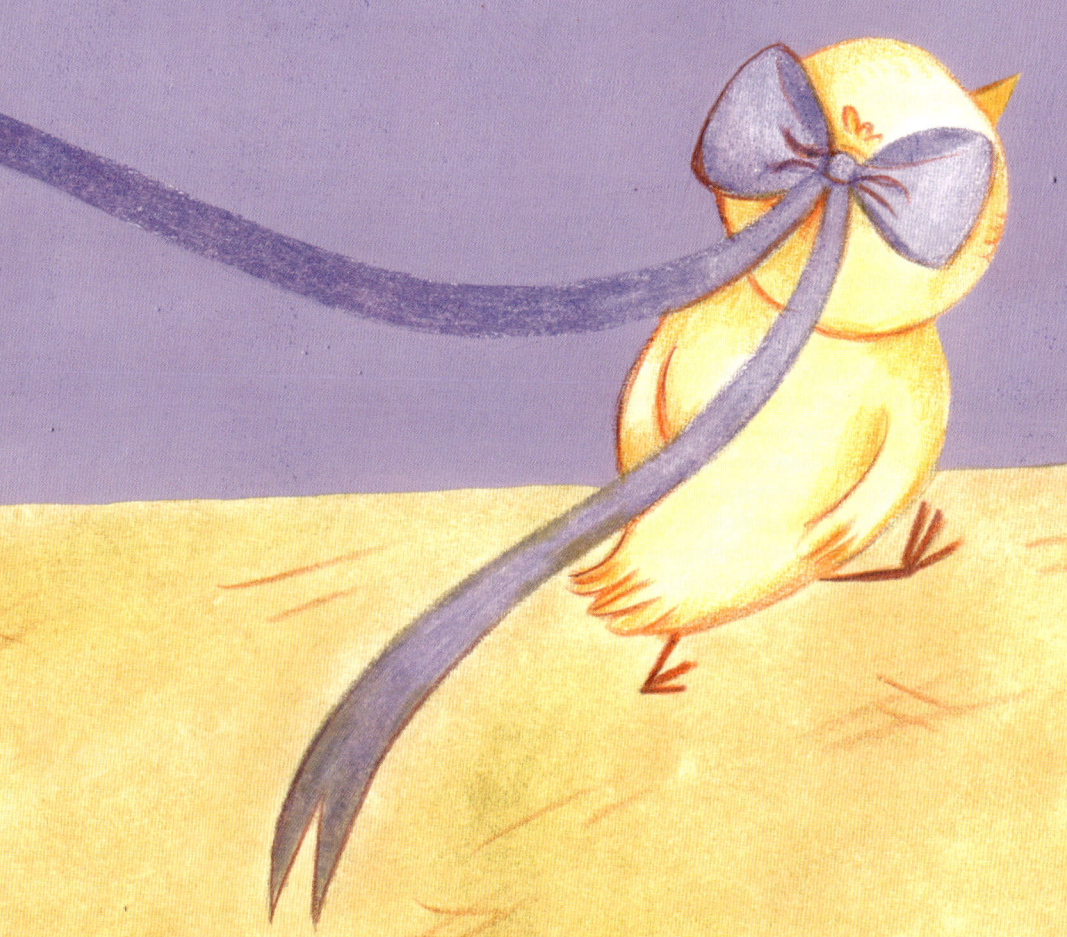

Maria Luisa Salcines and Maelia Salcines

Illustrated by Maria Ballarin

Chickadee peeked out from under her blanket.
She could hear her sisters playing outside her window.

"I need to get up. I need to get up," she said, but her arms
felt heavy. Her legs, too. She felt gloomy and blue.

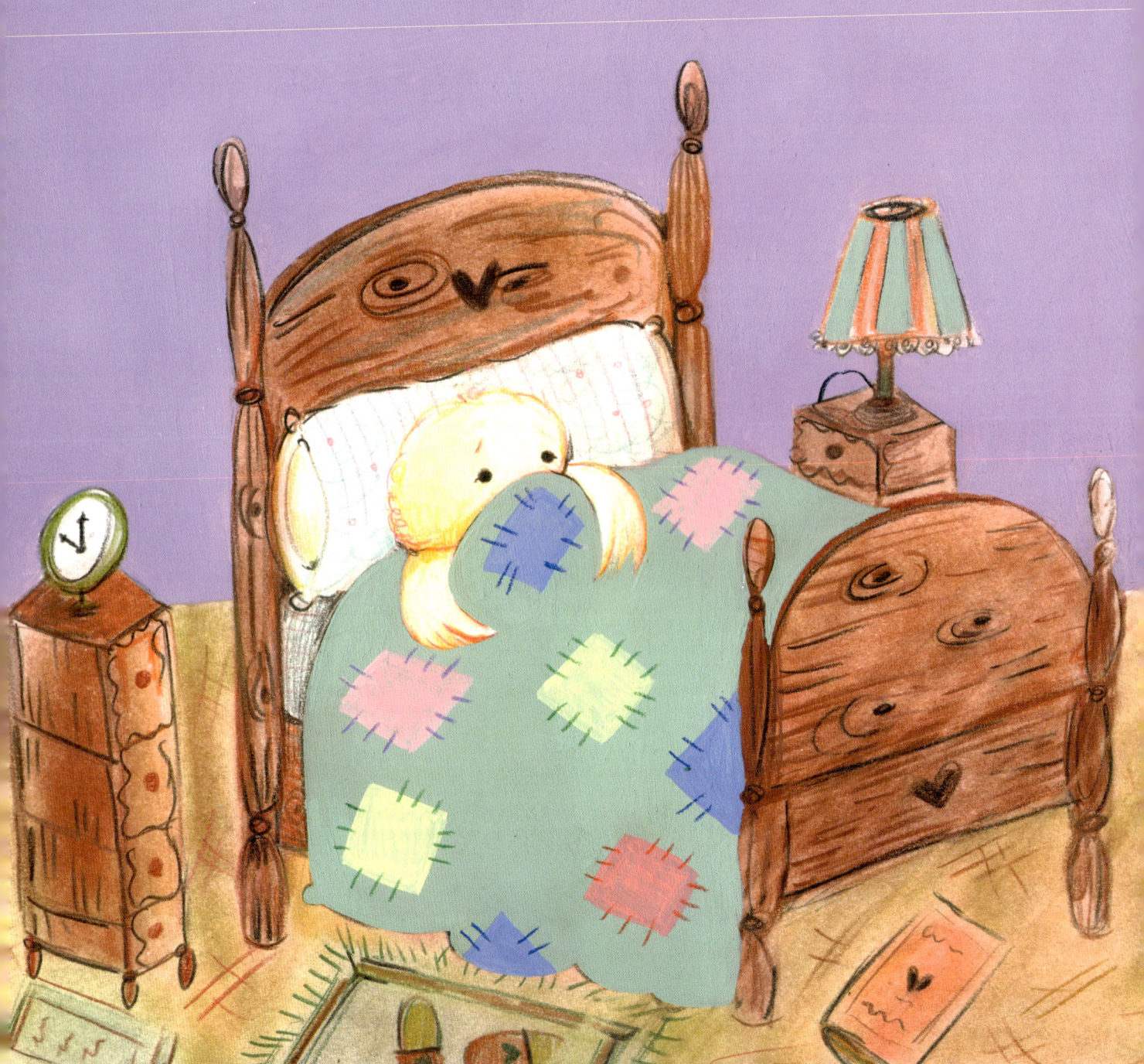

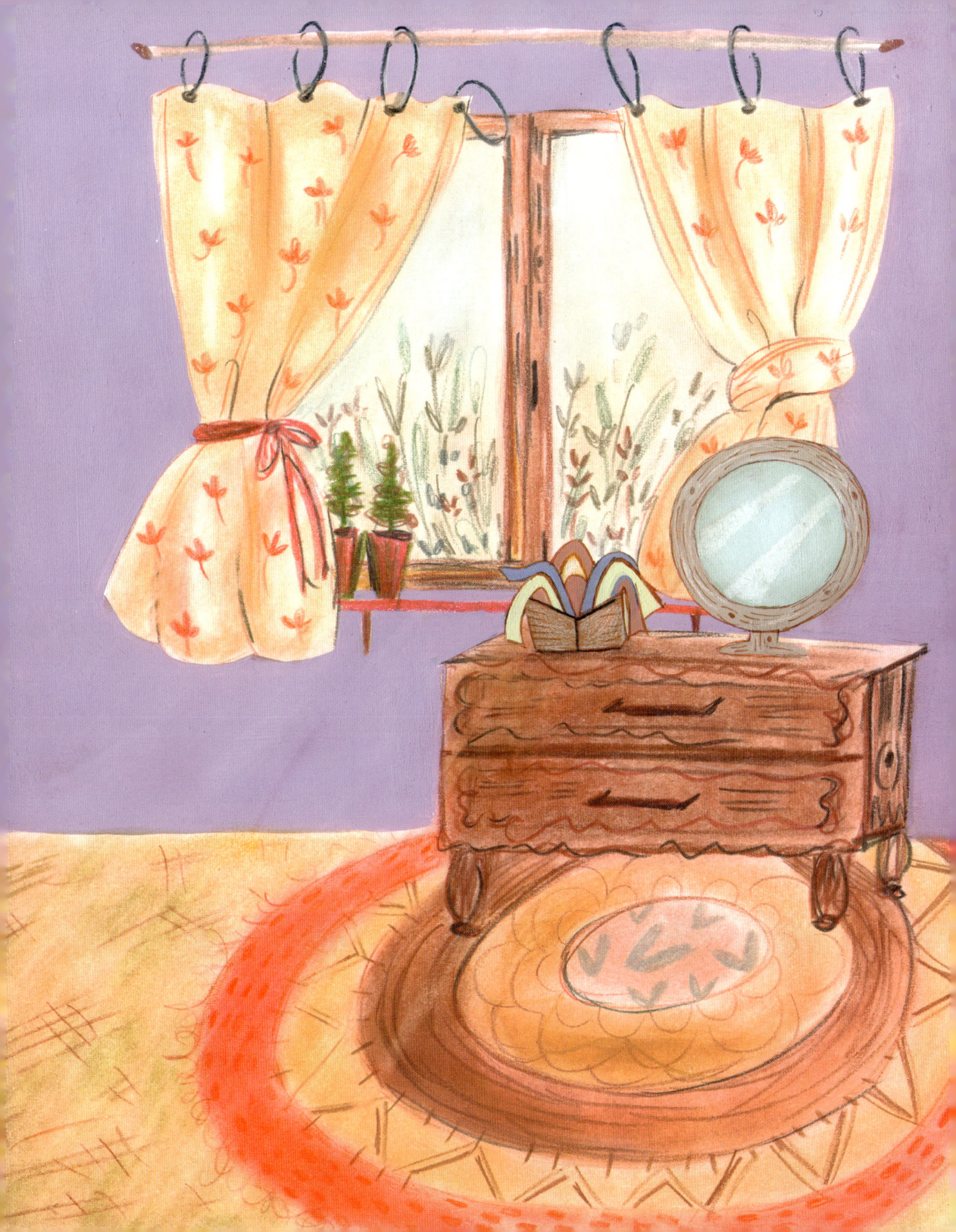

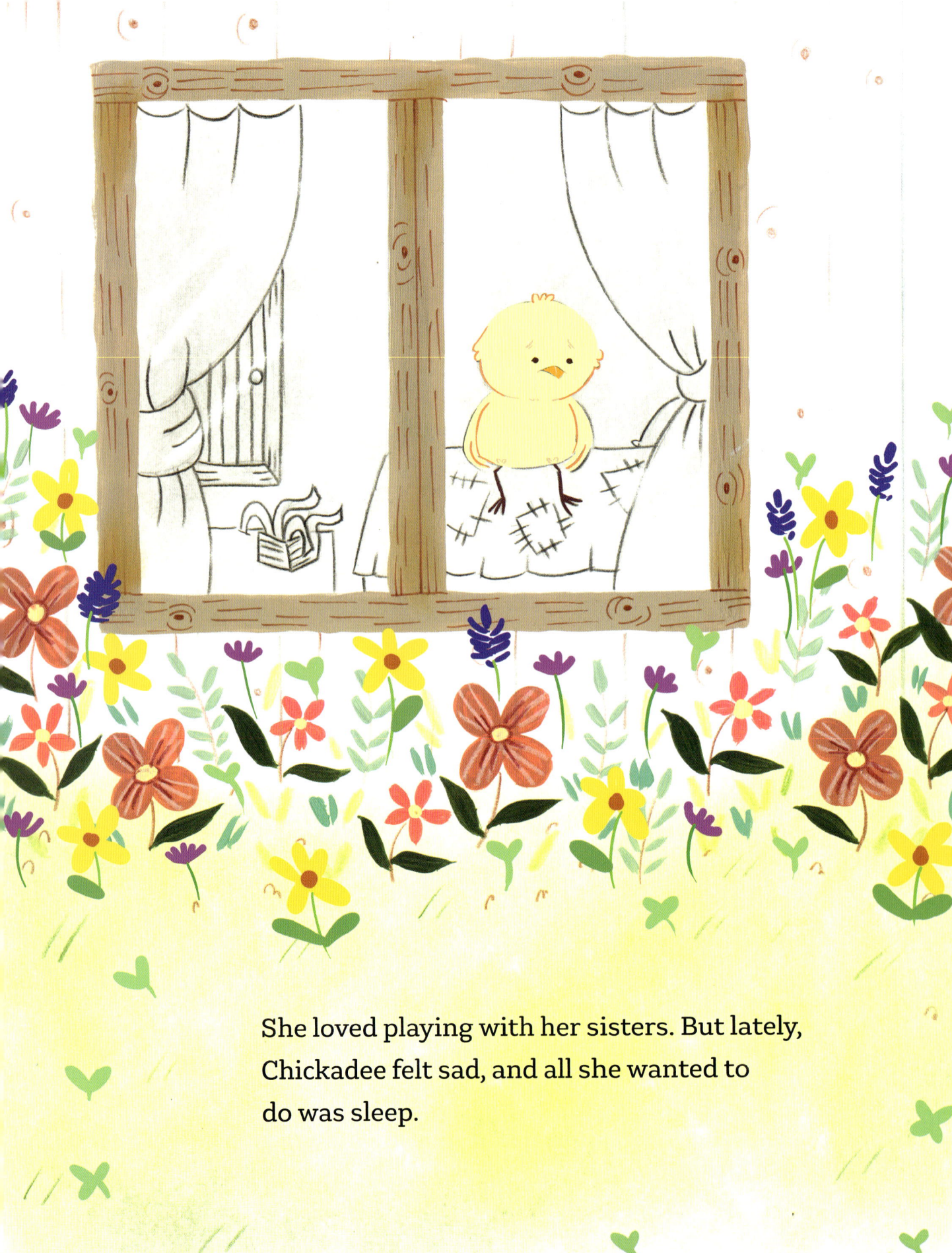

She loved playing with her sisters. But lately, Chickadee felt sad, and all she wanted to do was sleep.

Chickadee could hear her sisters laughing
outside, and she wanted to go out and join them.

"I CAN DO IT. I CAN DO IT,"

she said as she threw off the covers and got out of bed.

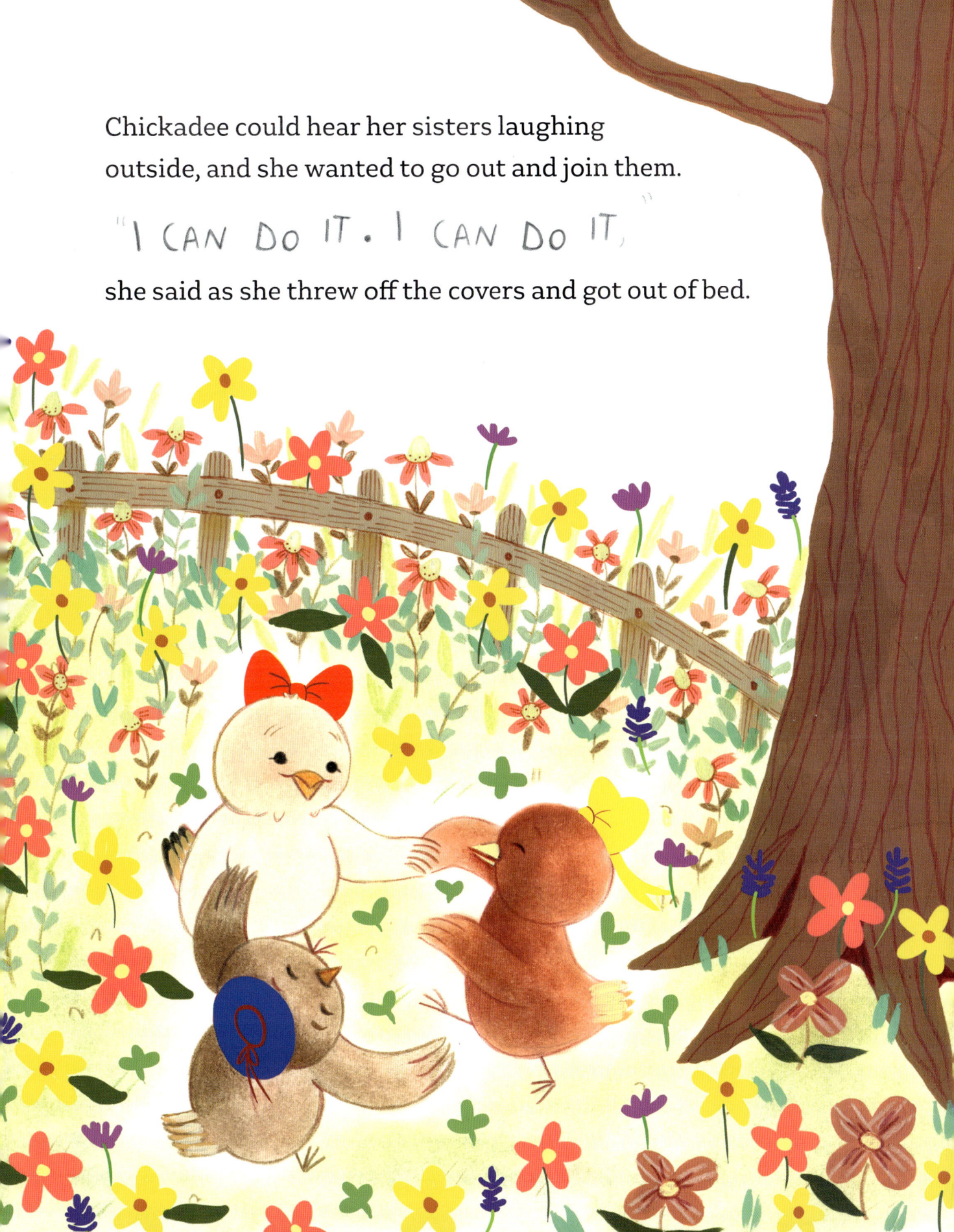

She ruffled her feathers and put on her favorite lavender bow.

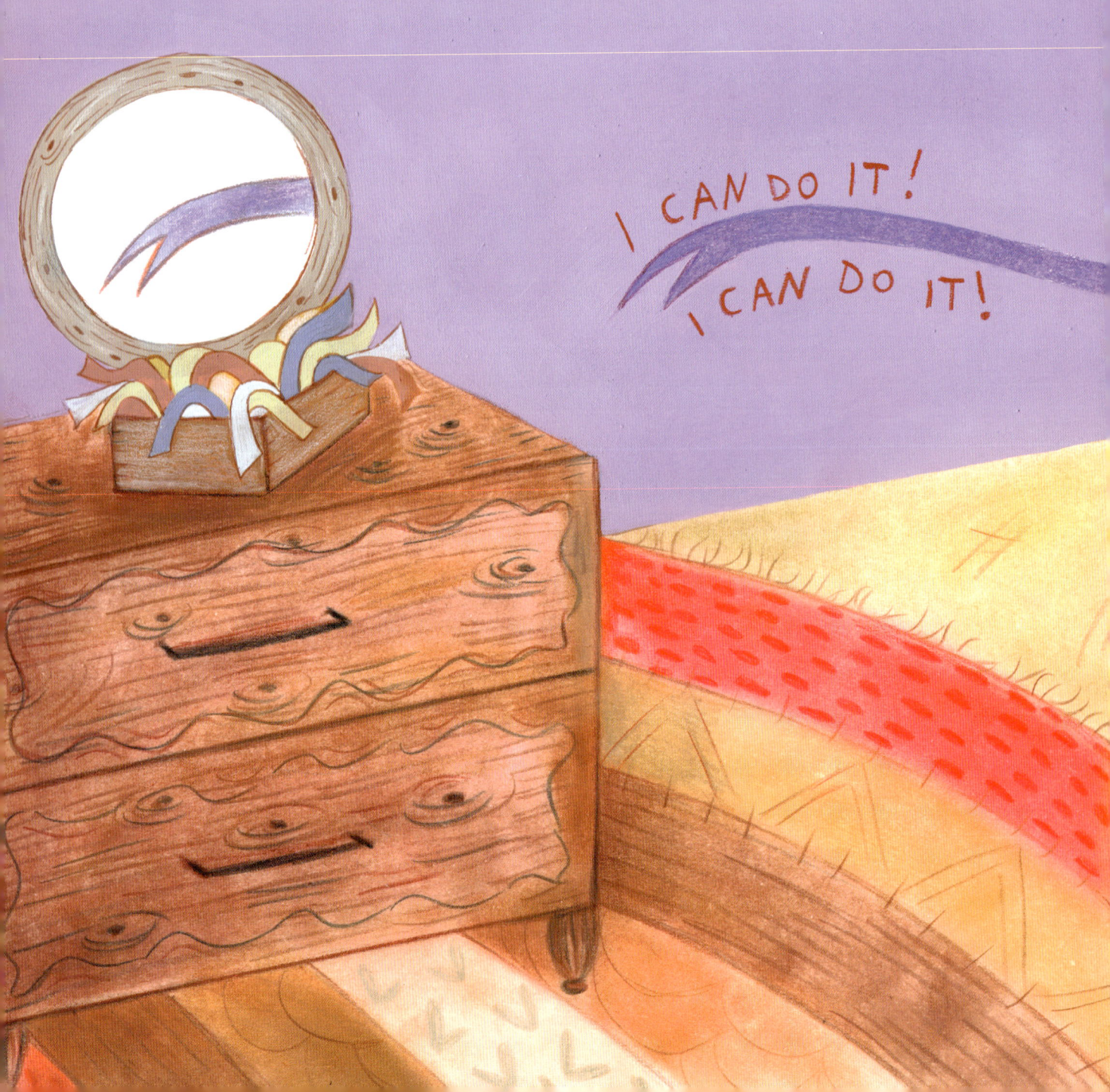

I CAN DO IT!
I CAN DO IT!

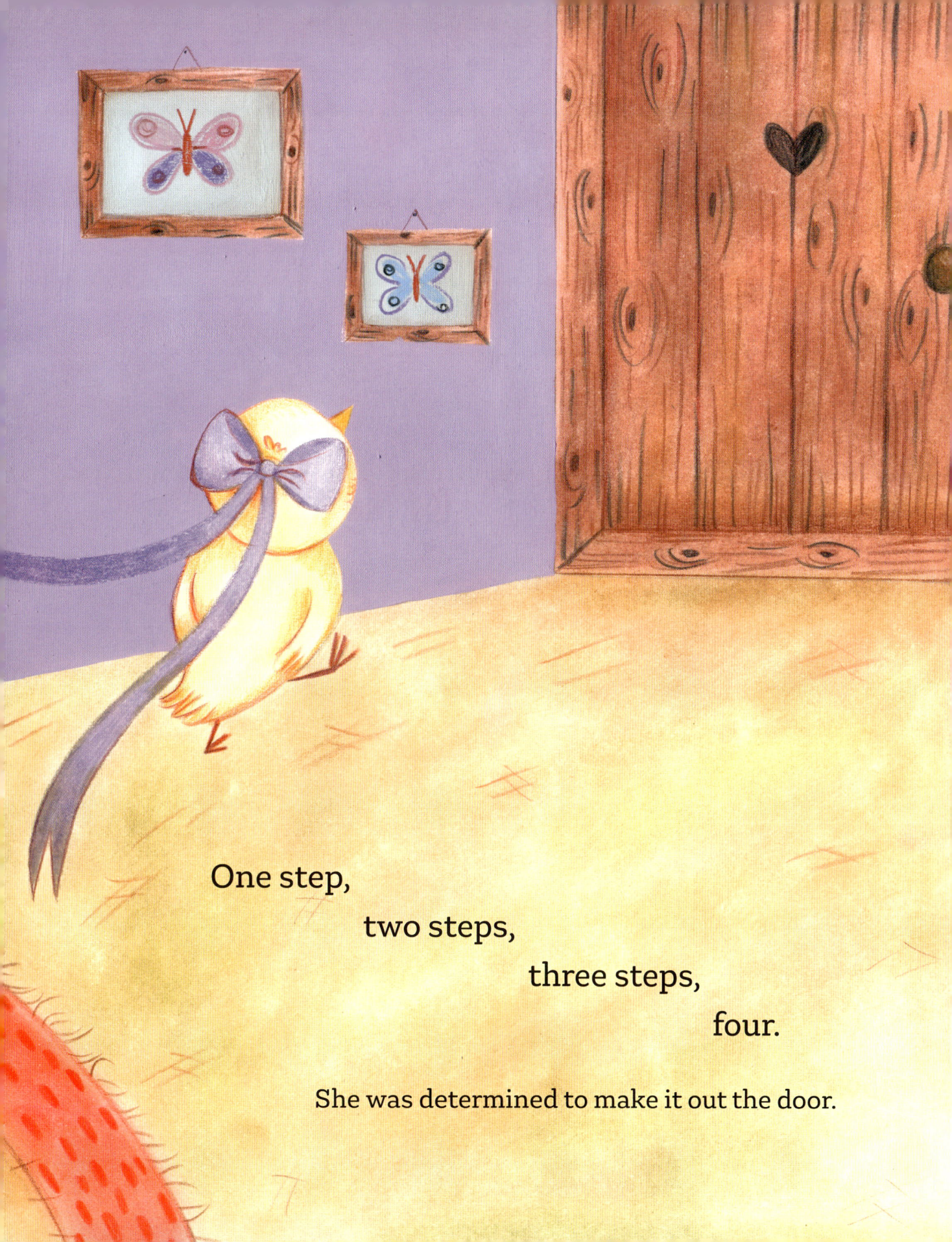

One step,

two steps,

three steps,

four.

She was determined to make it out the door.

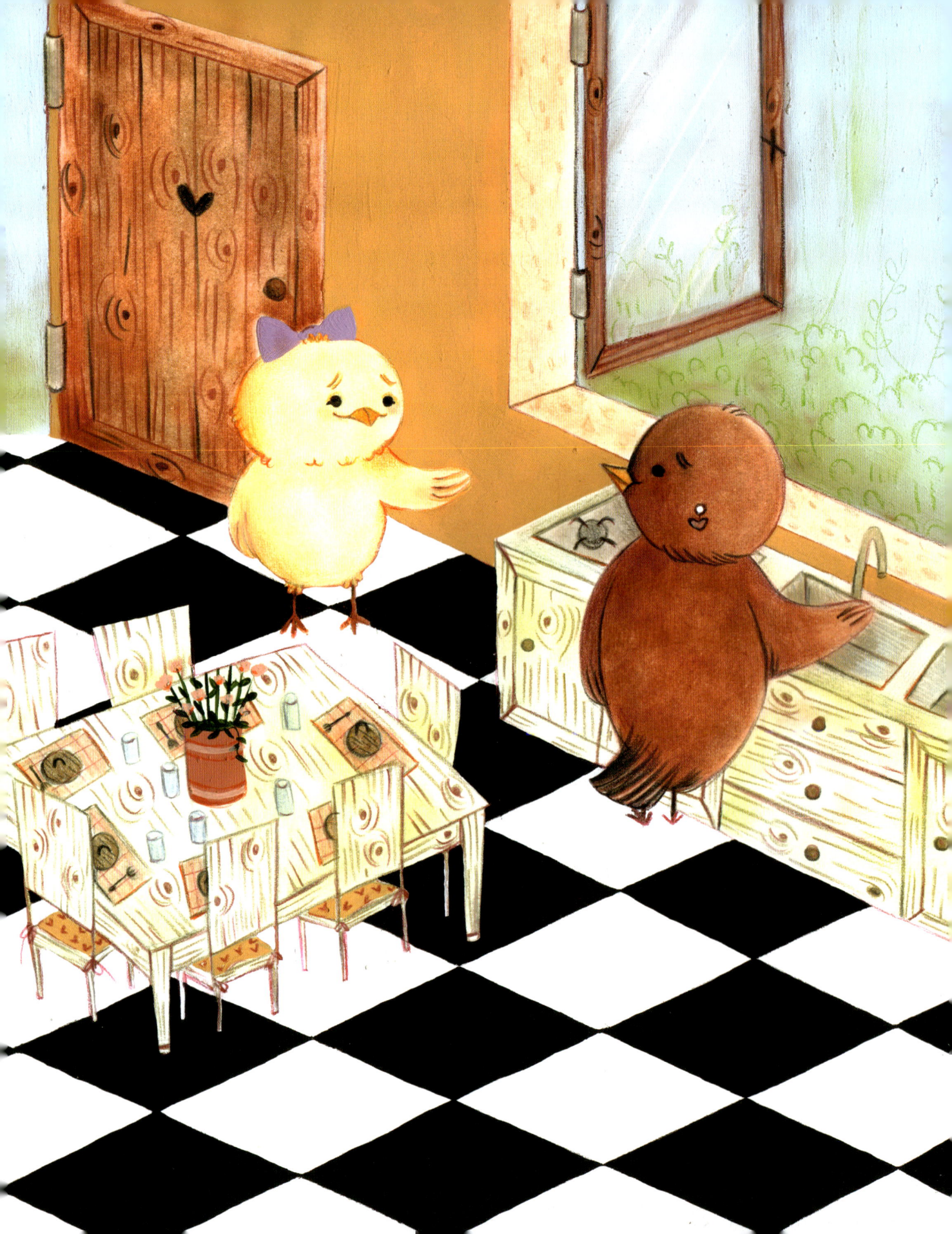

"Where are you going?" Mama asked as Chickadee walked through the kitchen toward the back door.

"Outside," Chickadee answered.

"Not until you eat breakfast and take your pills," Mama said.

"I'm not hungry!" Chickadee cried, tears gushing out of her eyes.

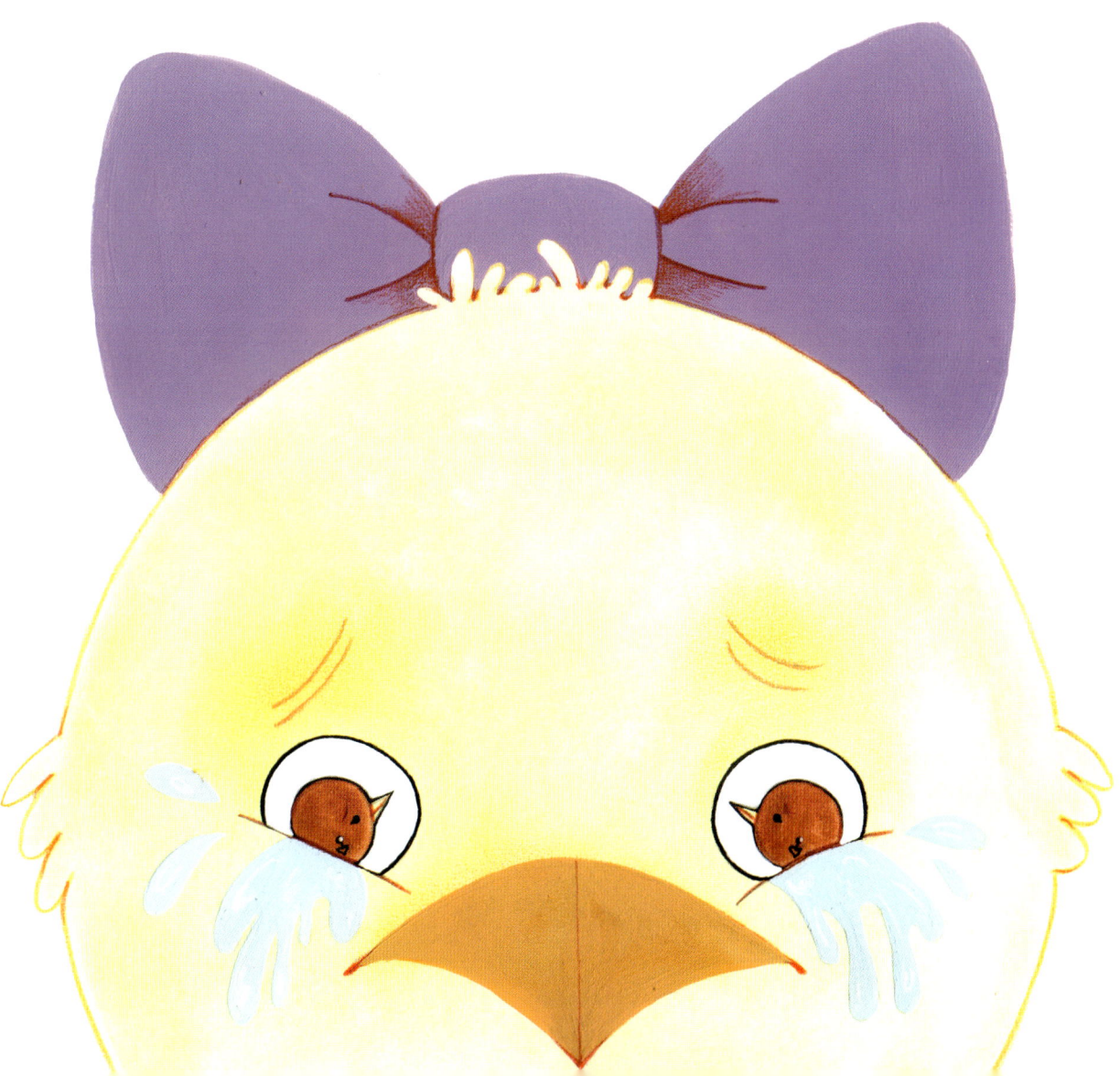

"Come here, sweetie," Mama said.

Chickadee dragged her feet on the floor:
One step, two steps, three steps, four.

"I made your favorite fluffy pancakes topped with strawberries
and slathered in maple syrup," Mama said.

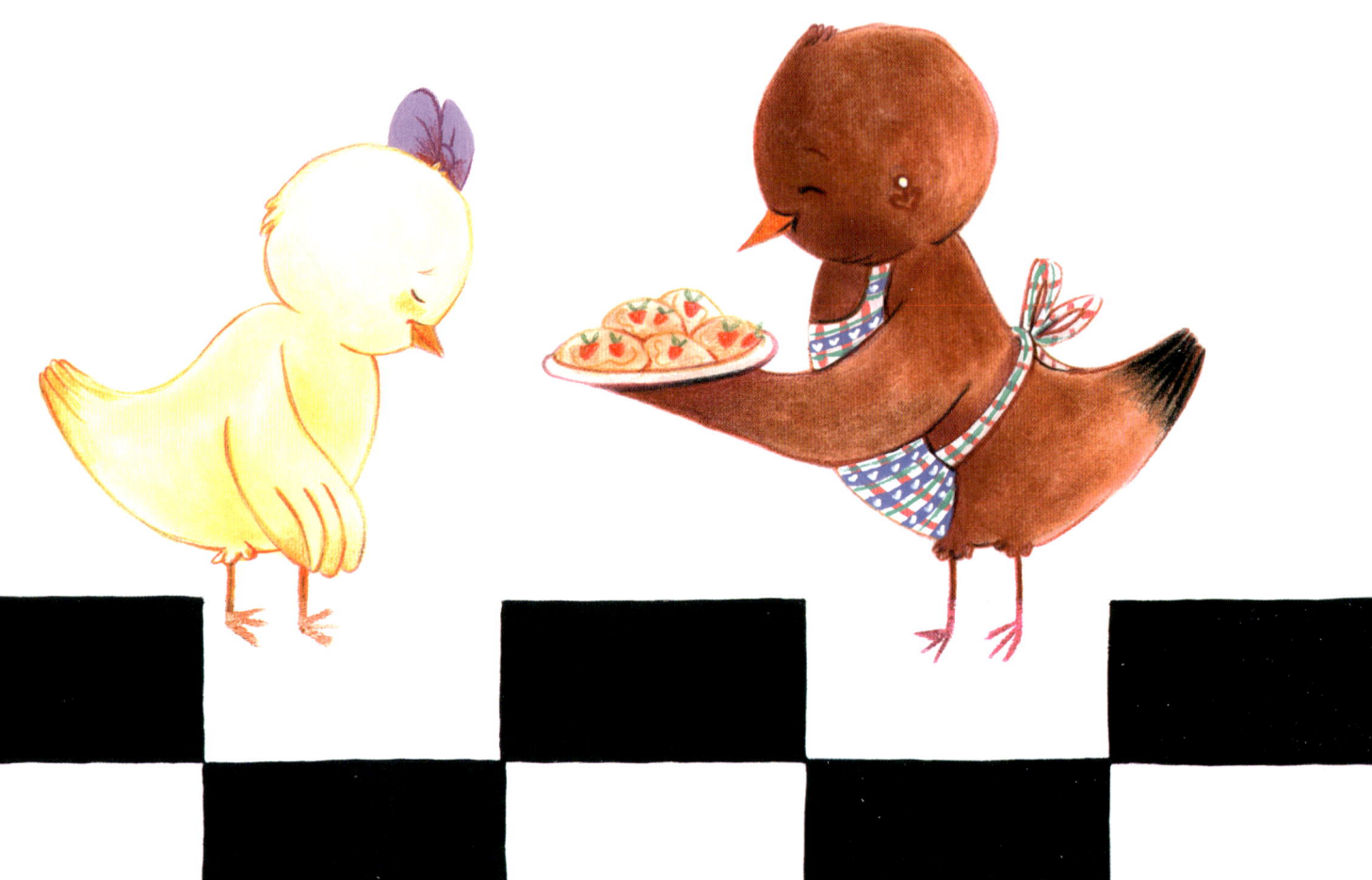

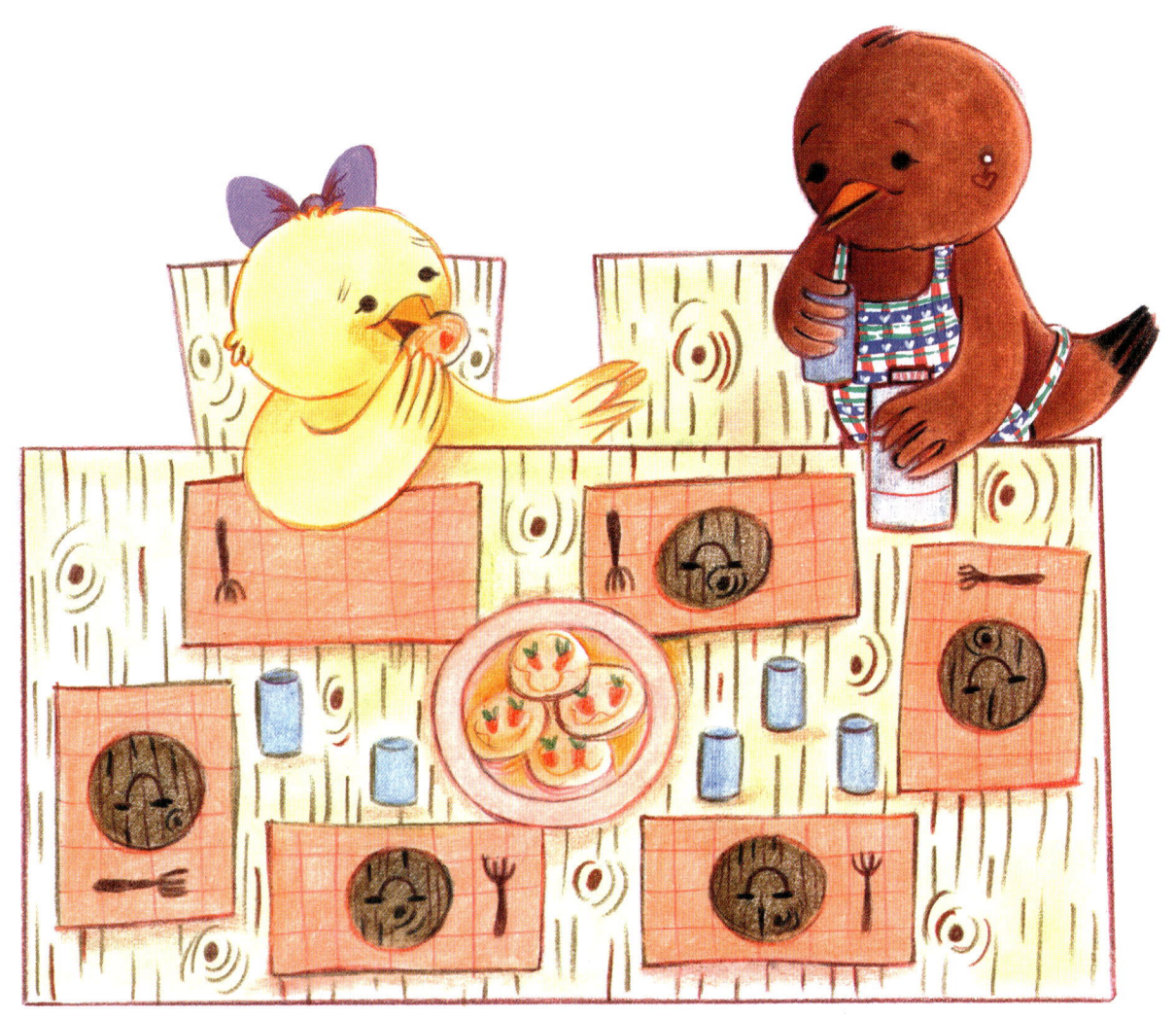

"It looks delicious," Chickadee said.
And she sat down and took:

One bite, two bites, three bites, four.

"Thank you, Mama," she said. "I'm sorry I yelled at you."

Sometimes when Chickadee doesn't feel good, she says mean things to those she loves, but she always apologizes and tries to do better.

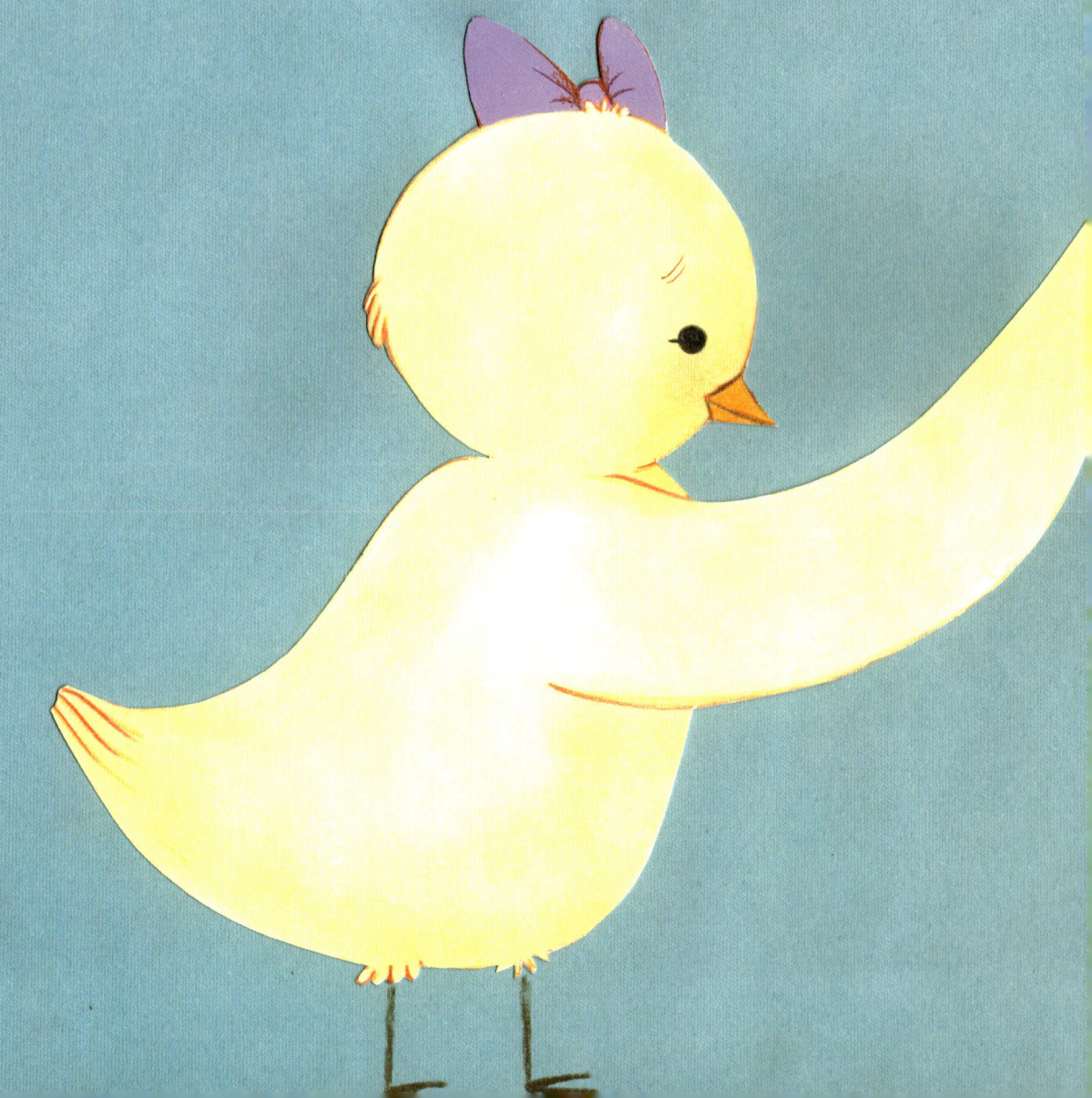

"It's okay, Chickadee. I love you even when you're grumpy."

"I'm going to go play now," Chickadee said. Taking:

One step,

two steps,

three steps,

four…

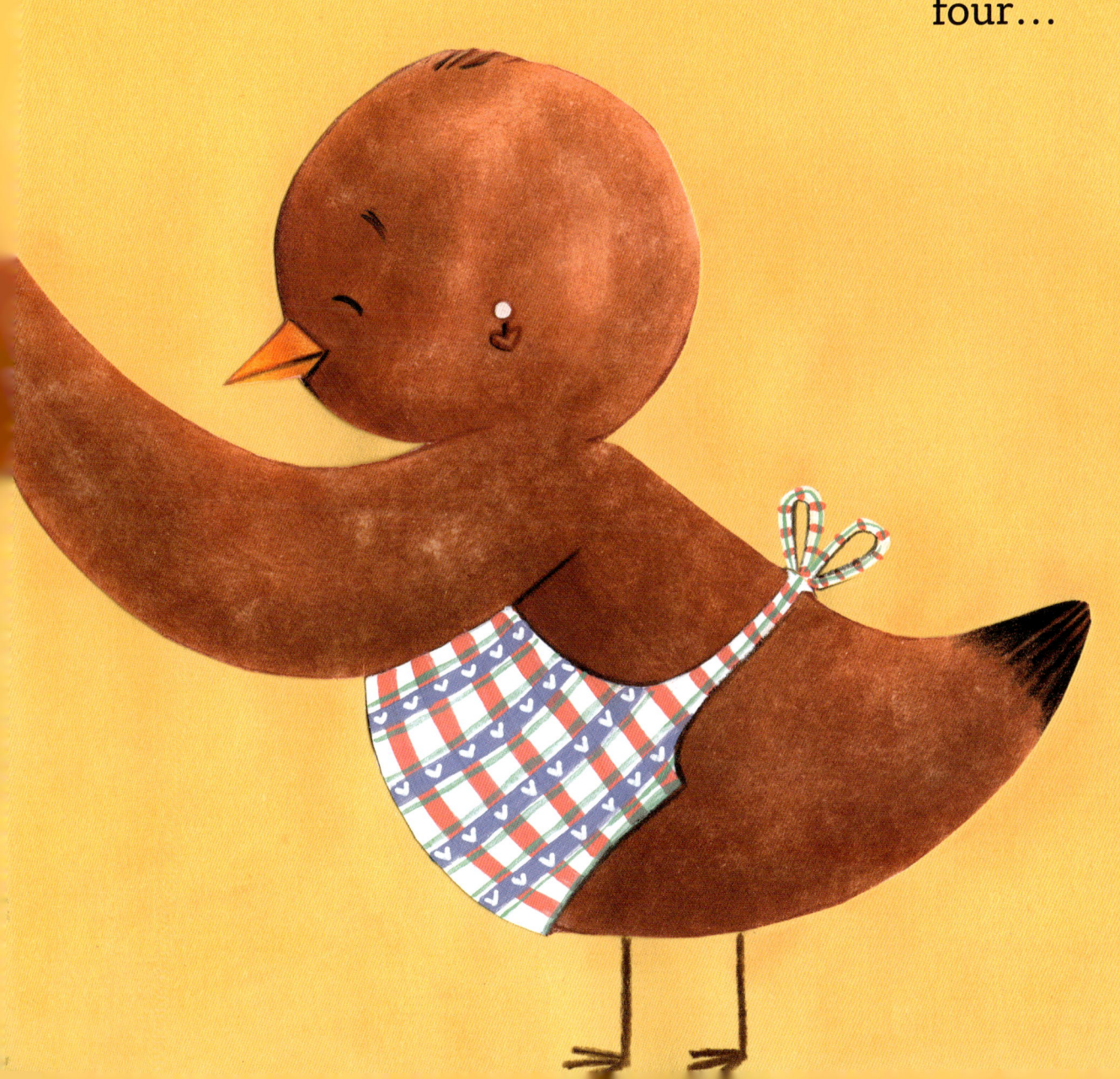

Taking her pills makes her feel different, and she wonders what her friends would think if they knew.

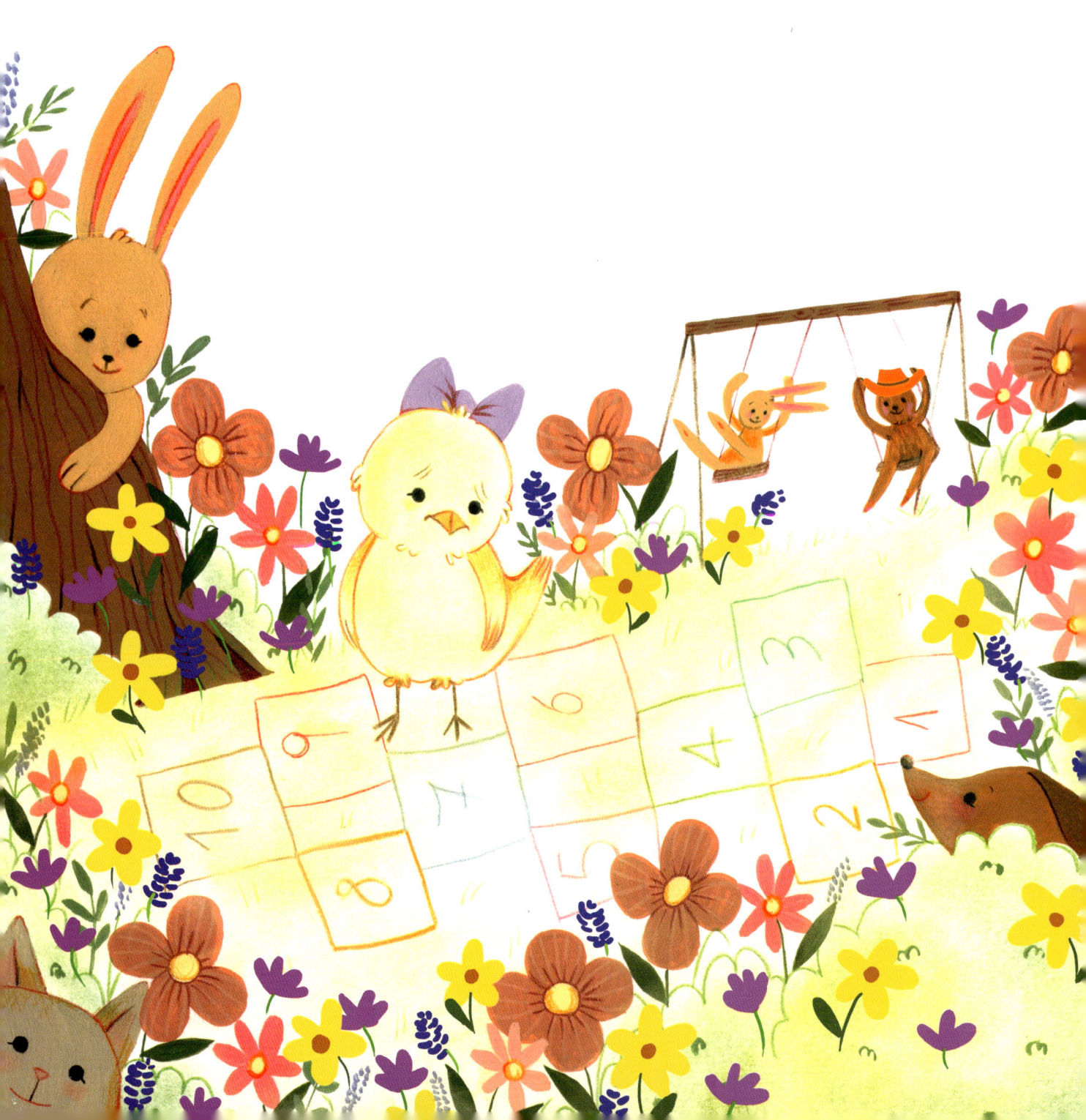

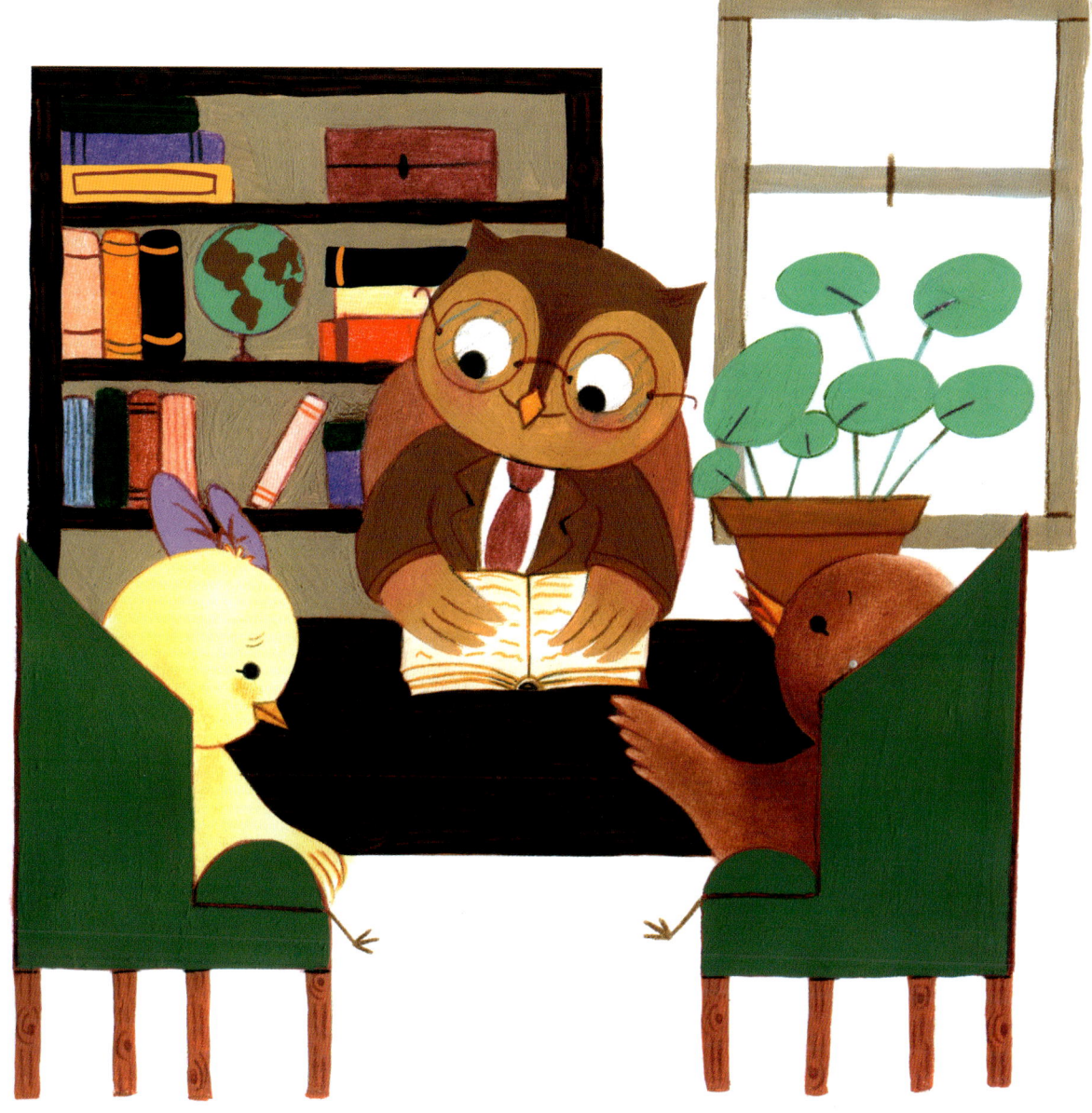

Chickadee started taking her pills after visiting
her therapist. She'd been feeling sad more and more
and had lost interest in things she loved, like playing
outside. Her therapist explained this was because
of depression and that with treatment, she could
start to feel better.

"I know taking medicine isn't fun," Mama said,
 handing her the pills and glass of water.

"But sometimes we all need to take medicine to feel better."

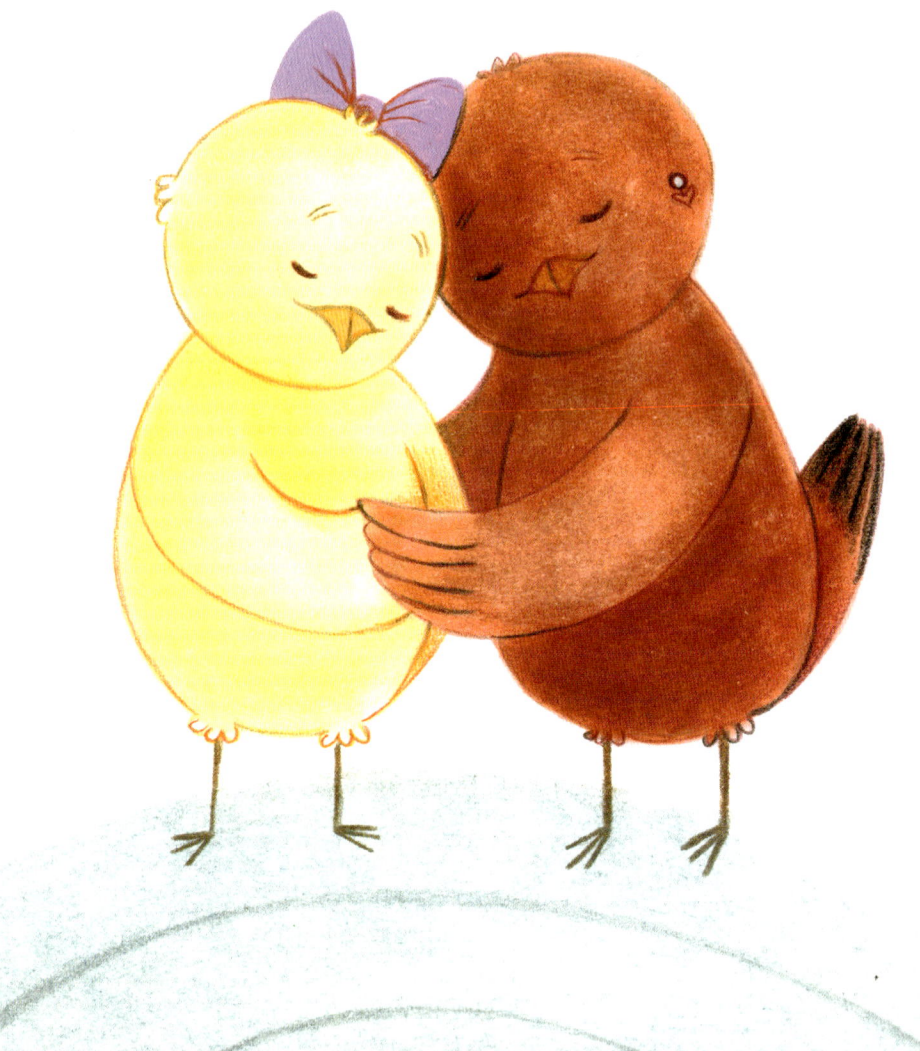

Chickadee took the pills, gave Mama a quick hug, and walked toward the door.

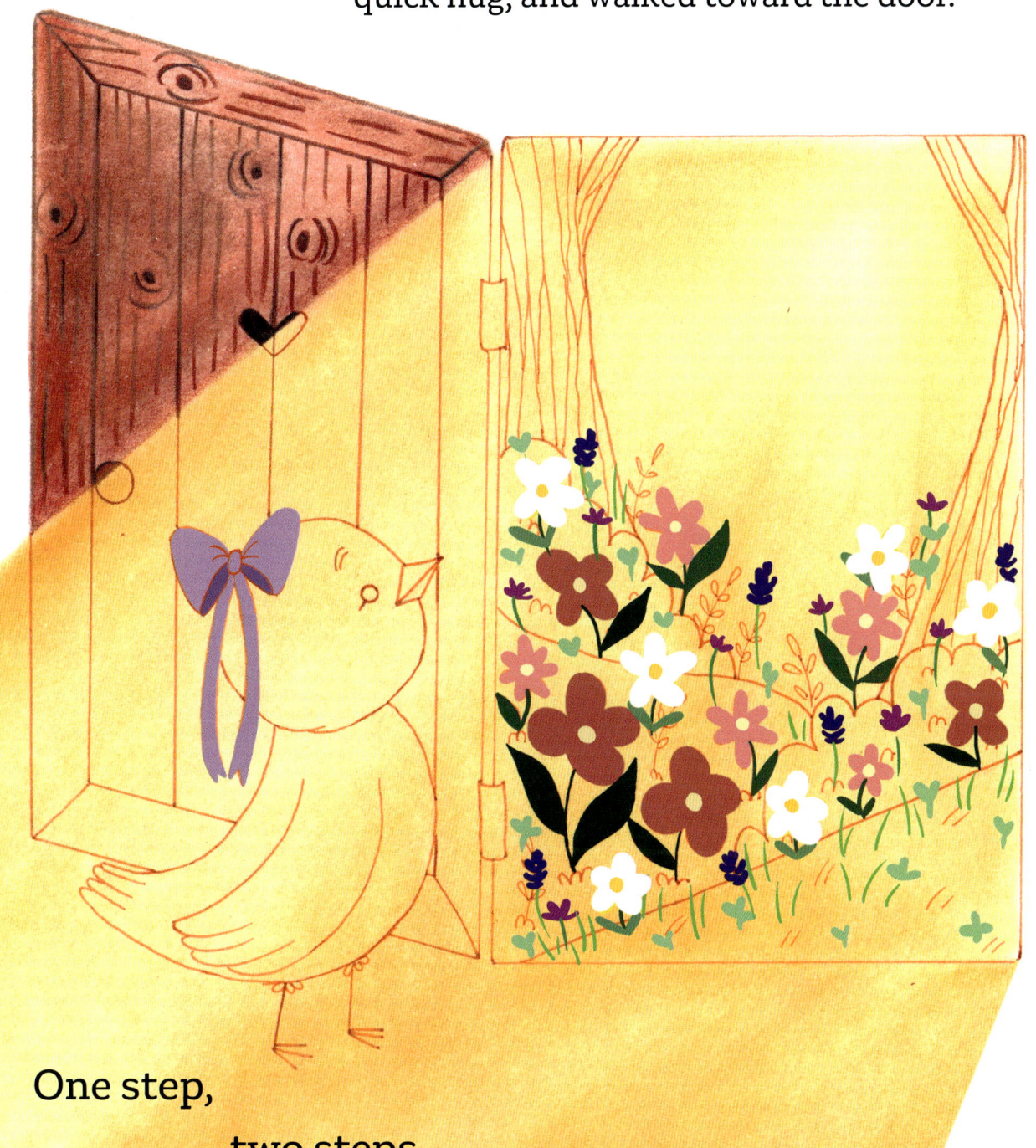

One step,

two steps,

three steps,

four...

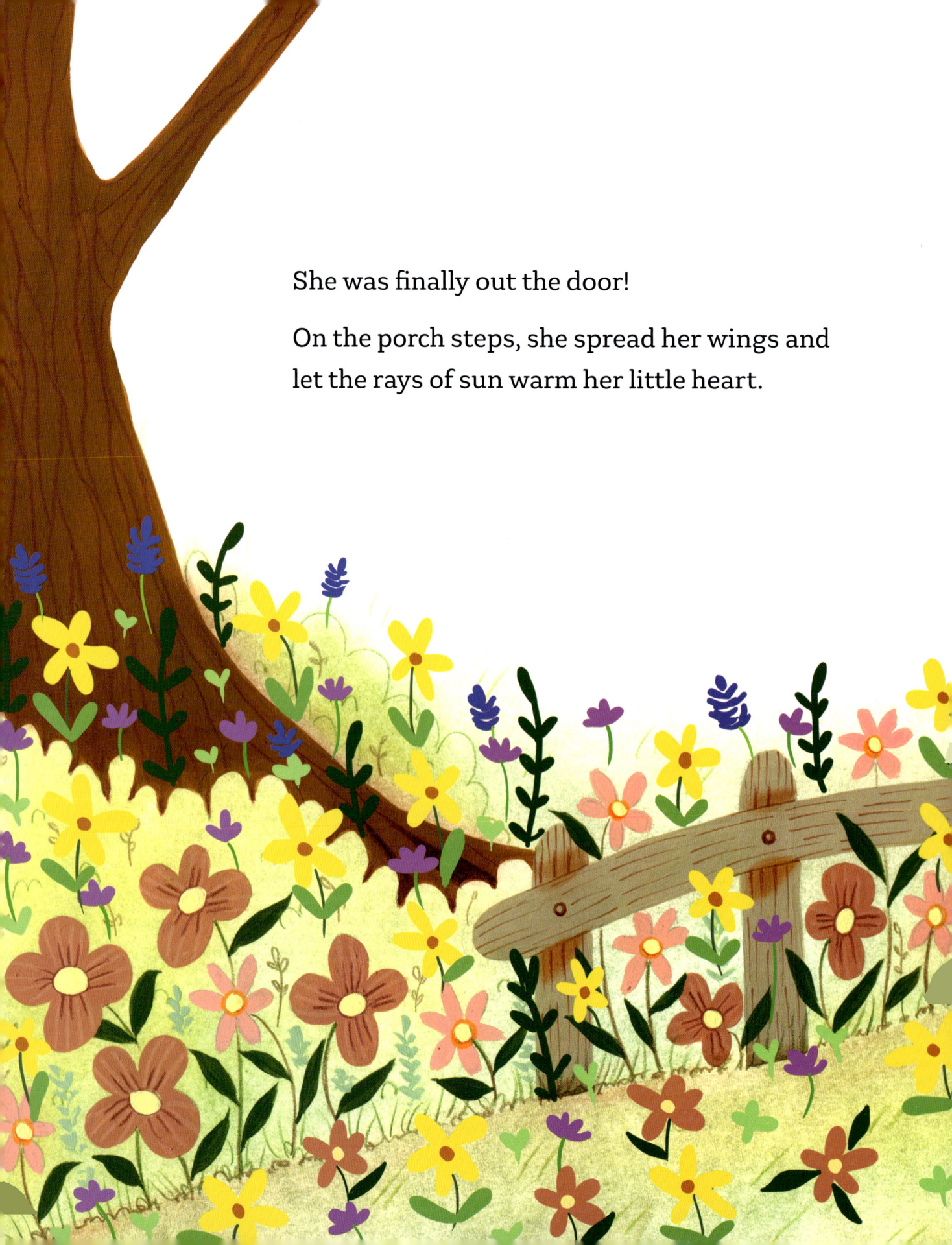

She was finally out the door!

On the porch steps, she spread her wings and let the rays of sun warm her little heart.

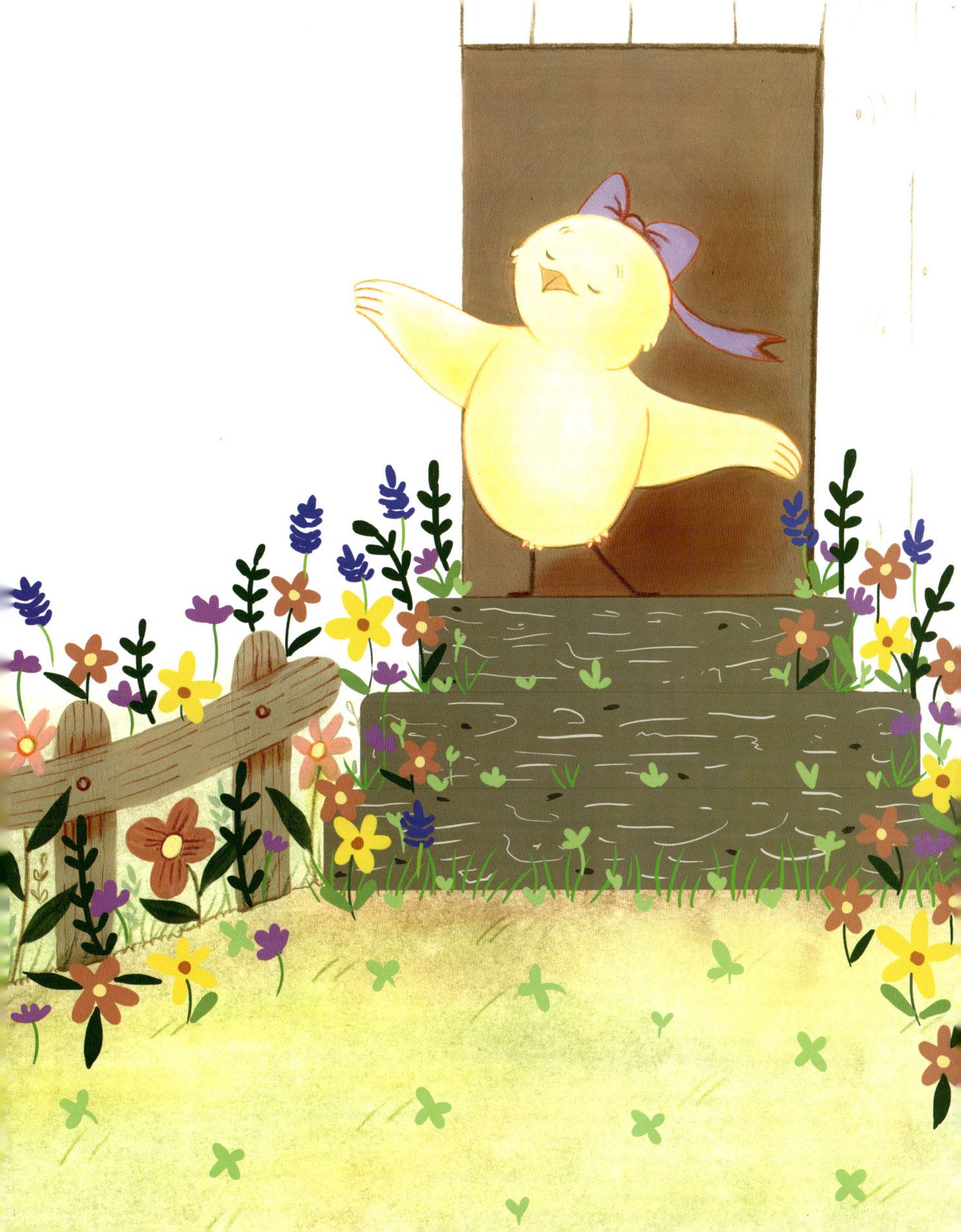

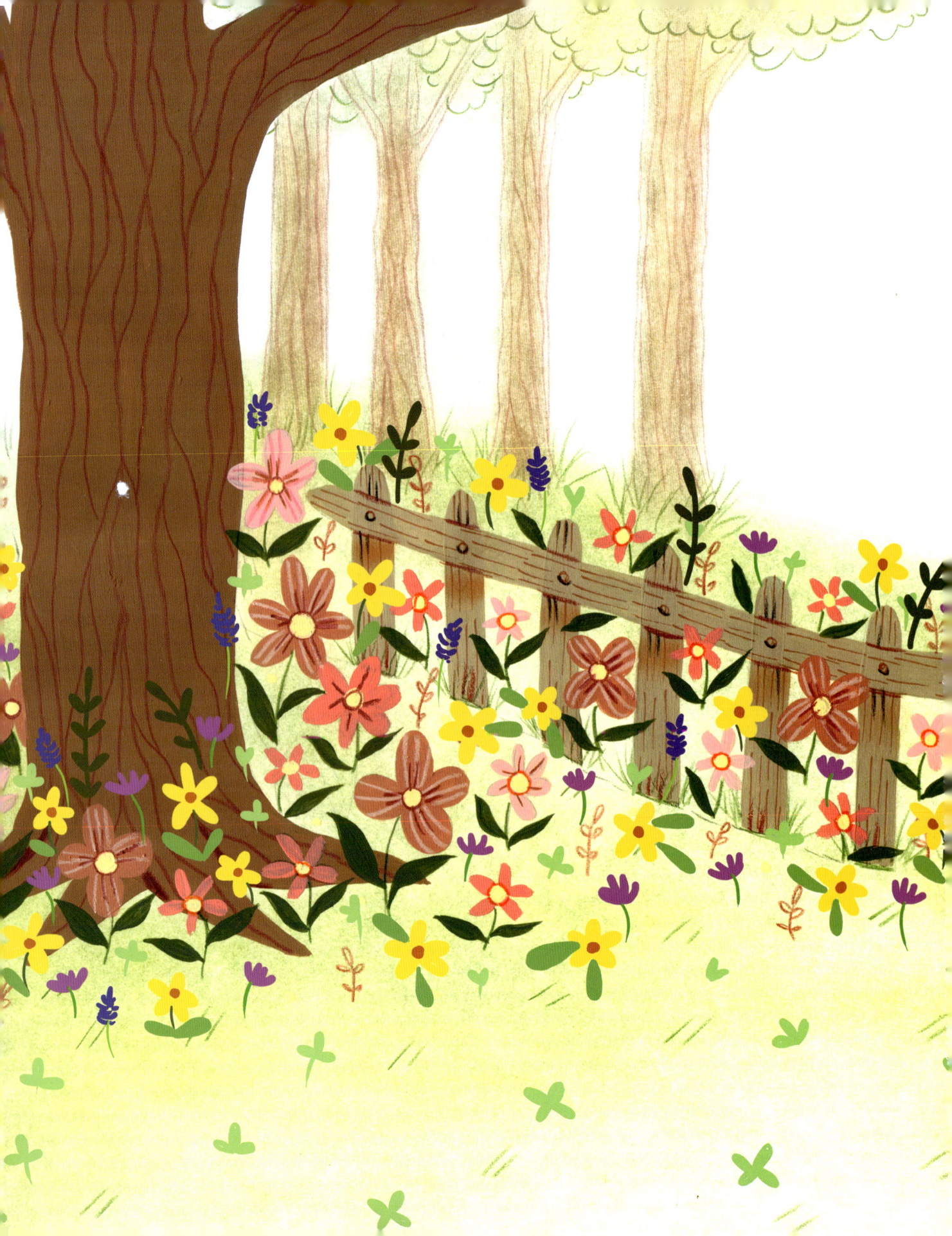

All she has to do is take:

One step,

two steps,

three steps,

at a time.

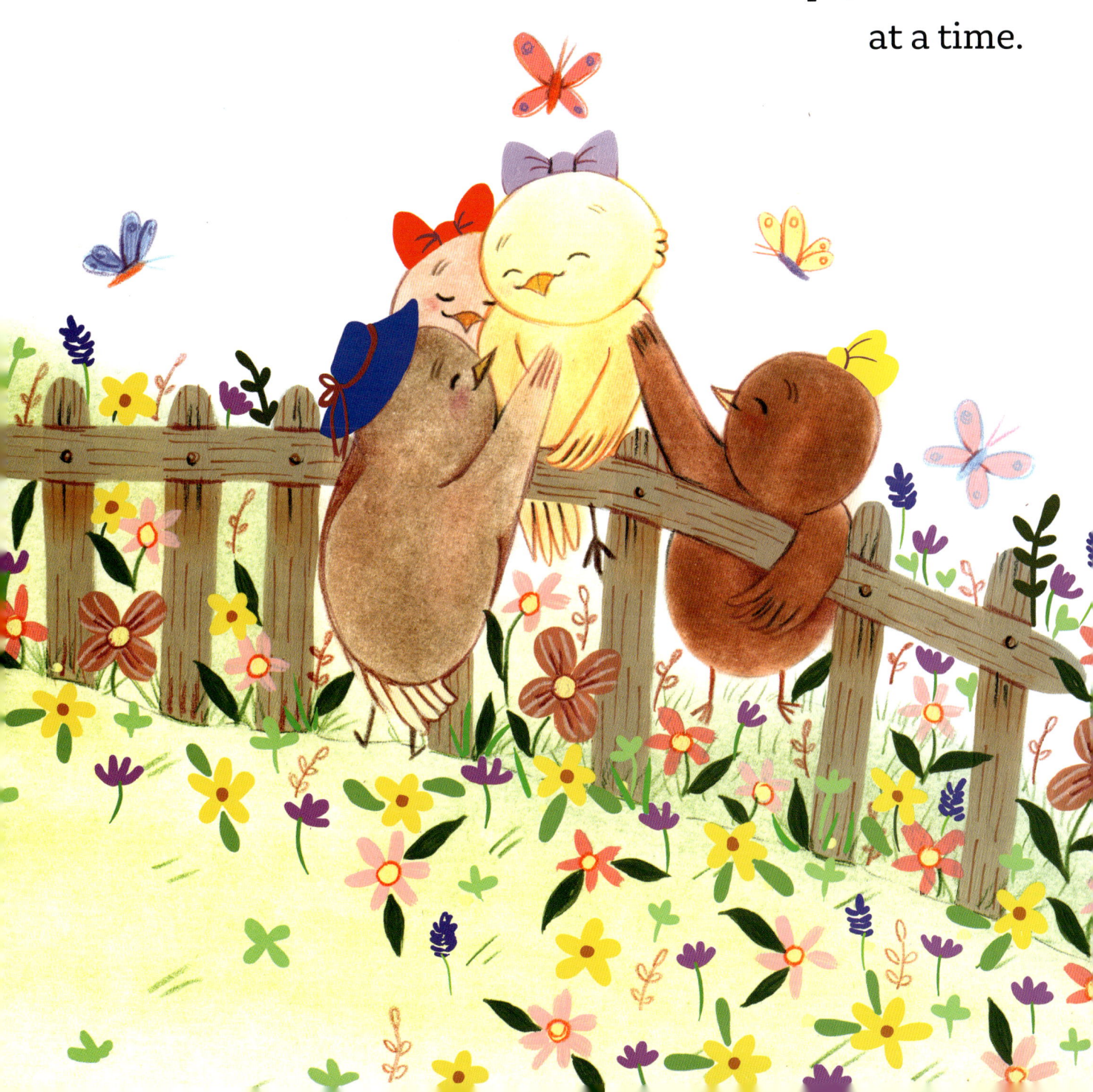

ABOUT THE AUTHORS

Maria Luisa Salcines and Maelia Salcines know firsthand how difficult dealing with depression can be. During her freshman year at St. Edward's University, Maelia was diagnosed with anxiety and depression. She spent the next two years learning to understand and cope with her diagnoses. It was during her on-stage question at her first pageant in which she won Miss Rio Grande Valley USA 2019 that she was asked, "What do you feel is your greatest accomplishment?" Her answer, which surprised her family and close friends who were the only ones who knew about her illness, was, "I think my greatest accomplishment is overcoming my anxiety and depression. It's been a long journey and very hard, but I am so thankful for the experience because it has made me the woman that I am today." Speaking publicly about her struggles was the first step toward accepting what she had experienced as a gift and making addressing mental illness her life purpose. Maelia is a senior at South Texas College pursuing a bachelor of applied technology in technology management. She is the co-founder of Mental Monarchs Inc., a nonprofit organization and blog dedicated to spreading awareness and knowledge in hope to end the stigma of mental illness. Based in South Texas, Mental Monarchs raises money to help pay for counseling services for individuals who cannot afford it. Maelia is the current Miss Heart of Texas USA 2020 and was Miss Rio Grande Valley USA 2019. Her passion is speaking and writing about mental illness.

www.mentalmonarchs.com

@maeliatx   @mentalmonarchs

Maria Luisa Salcines is a freelance writer whose work has appeared in newspapers and magazines. She is the author of *Little Things Remembered*, a collection of stories on love, parenting, and cultural identity, and co-author of *Maggie's Visit to the Playroom*, *Play Time for Molly*, *Matt's in Trouble Again*, and *Matt Otra Vez en Problemas*. These children's books discuss play therapy, filial therapy, and school counseling. Maria Luisa is a certified parent educator and parent coach with The Academy of Parenting Education and Coaching in Redirecting Children's Behavior and Redirecting for a Cooperative Classroom.

www.marialsalcines | www.familylifeandfindinghappy

@mlsalcinespoweroffamily   FamilyLifeAndFindingHappy

LETTER TO PARENTS

Family discussions about mental illness will encourage children to be open about their feelings and help them better handle their mental health as they get older. It is important that parents and educators talk to children about mental health. Normalizing the topic will help reduce the risk of children isolating or withdrawing from their loved ones in order to hide what they are feeling, which usually exacerbates and worsens mental health issues.

Most children will go through periods when they feel sad and hopeless. Most fears and worries appear at different stages of a child's development. However, when a child has extreme forms of sadness and fears, it may be due to a mental illness.

According to the Center for Disease Control and Prevention, "One out of six children aged 2-8 years has a mental, behavioral, or developmental disorder and 3.2% of children aged 3-17 years (approximately 1.9 million) have diagnosed depression. For youth ages 10-24 years, suicide is among the leading causes of death."

Recognizing symptoms and early diagnosis is key for the success of a child with a mental illness. If you are concerned with your child's mental health, consult your child's doctor. Talk to those close to your child (teacher, relatives, and caregiver) and ask if they have noticed changes in his or her behavior. Ask your child's doctor to refer you to services that can screen and treat mental disorders.

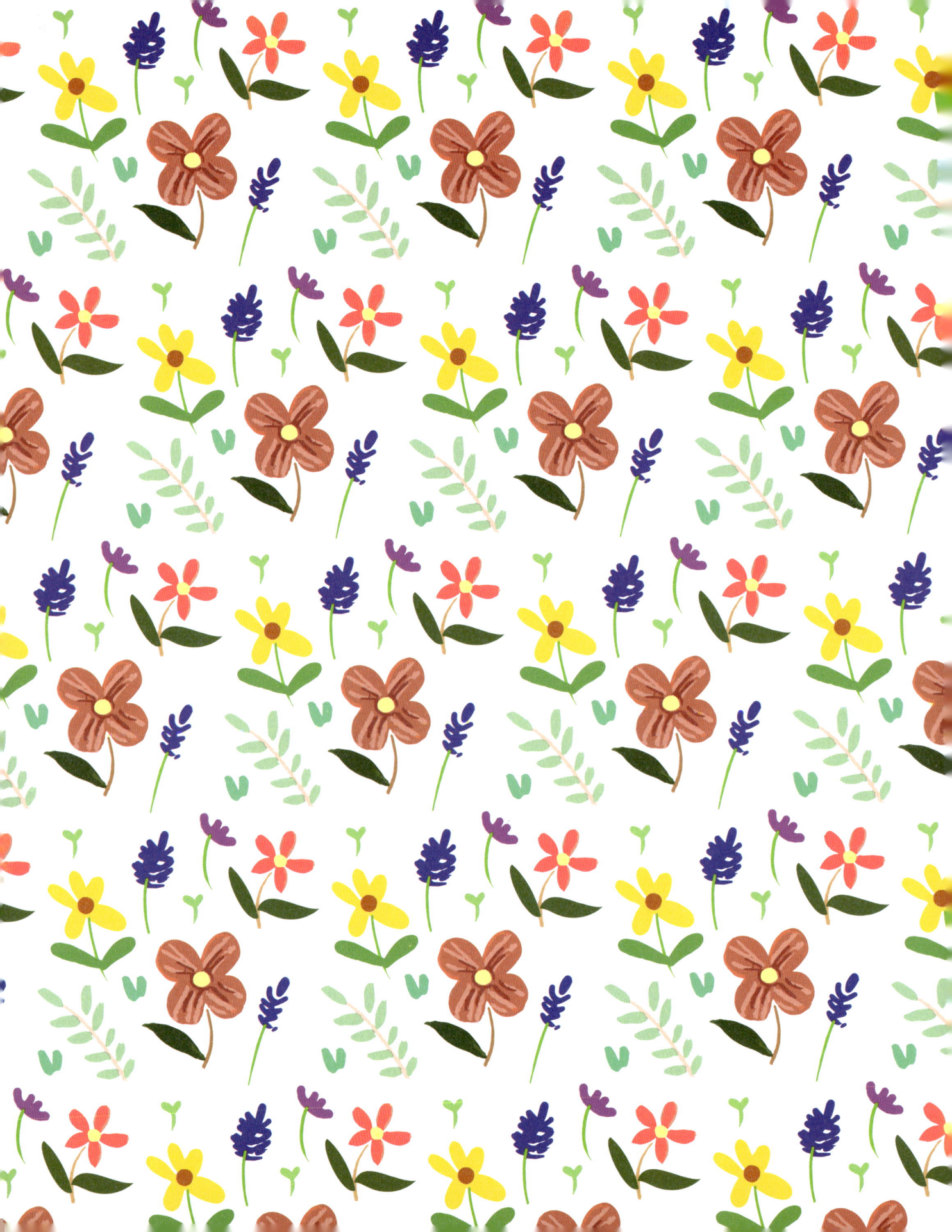